# The Glucose Code:

## The Extraordinary Force Of Stabilizing Your Blood Sugar Level

By

## William T. Walker

# Disclaimer

# Table Of Contents

# Introduction

The structure of glucose has six carbon atoms and the chemical formula $C_6H_{12}O_6$. It is necessary to fuel both aerobic and anaerobic cellular respiration and is a common source of energy for all living things. Glucose frequently enters the body in isometric structures like galactose and fructose (monosaccharides), lactose and sucrose (disaccharides), or starch (polysaccharides). When we fast, the excess glucose that is stored in our bodies is released as glycogen, a glucose polymer. Through the process of gluconeogenesis, glucose can also be produced from the byproducts of the breakdown of fat and protein. Taking into account how crucial glucose is for homeostasis, it is nothing unexpected that there are plenty of hotspots for it.

When glucose is in the body, it goes through the blood and to energy-requiring tissues. There, glucose is separated in a progression of biochemical responses delivering energy as ATP.

The ATP obtained from these cycles is utilized to fuel every energy-requiring process in the body. In eukaryotes, most energy comes from vigorous (oxygen-requiring) processes, which start with a particle of glucose.

The glucose is separated first through the anaerobic course of glycolysis, prompting the creation of some ATP and pyruvate final result. Pyruvate undergoes reduction into lactate in anaerobic conditions. In high-impact conditions, the pyruvate can enter the citrus extract cycle to yield energy-rich electron transporters that assist with creating ATP at the electron transport chain.

# Chapter 1: What is Glucose and Why is it important?

Glucose is the fundamental kind of sugar in the blood and is the significant wellspring of energy for the body's cells. Glucose comes from the food varieties we eat or the body can make it from different substances. Glucose is brought to the cells through the circulatory system. A few chemicals, including insulin, control glucose levels in the blood. Glucose is otherwise called blood sugar. The body's framework should work appropriately. When our blood glucose levels are at their highest, it frequently goes unnoticed. At the point when the degree of glucose is high then you can feel the unfortunate working impacts.

## Anyway, what precisely is glucose?

It is a monosaccharide, i.e. the most straightforward type of sugar. This suggests that it only contains one sugar. Fructose, galactose, and ribose are instances of monosaccharides. It is one of the body's favored wellsprings of fuel as starches and fat.

Bread, organic products, vegetables, and dairy items are great wellsprings of glucose. Food is expected to deliver energy. Energy is expected to keep you alive. While it is fundamental, as such countless different things, it is best consumed with some restraint. Long-term harm can result from glucose levels that are unhealthy or out of control.

**For what reason is Glucose significant?**

- Every cell in the human body needs energy. To do this metabolic capabilities keep us alive. The brain, muscles, and a wide range of other body organs and tissues all rely heavily on glucose, a tiny, simple sugar.

- It is likewise a part of the body's greater underlying particles, like glycoproteins and glycolipids. These levels in the human body are firmly directed. Unusually high or low levels could cause huge outcomes. However, it has other negative effects that put lives in danger.

- The mind's energy needs are by and large met for the most part by glucose. Our mind requires a consistent stockpile of glucose because of its high energy requests and failure to hold it. Numerous frameworks exist in the body to forestall an enormous drop in glucose, in some cases known as hypoglycemia. However, brain function may begin to fail if this occurs.

- Cerebral pain, as well as dizziness and other conditions such as; disarray, absence of consideration, uneasiness, crabbiness, anxiety, slurred discourse, and unfortunate coordination are normal hypoglycemia cerebrum side effects. A sudden and significant drop in blood sugar can cause seizures and coma.

- Develops Muscle and Provides Energy Skeletal muscles typically contribute between 30 and 40 percent of the body's weight. However, this differs depending on sex, age, and wellness level.

During the physical action, the skeletal muscles consume a ton of glucose. In contrast to the brain, skeletal muscles store blood sugar as glycogen, which is quickly broken down to provide glucose when exercising.

- Serves as a Fuel for Tissues and Organs in the body, which make use of a high amount of fuels. Other fundamental organs and tissues, especially the cerebrum and skeletal muscles, use glucose as their essential or sole wellspring of energy. As well as other tissues and organs which includes; the eye's cornea, lens, and retina, as well as red and white blood cells. Even though the small intestine cells are in charge of transferring glucose from meals into the bloodstream. It to a great extent involves glutamine as a wellspring of energy. This opens up additional glucose for organs and tissues that are more sugar-subordinate.

# Chapter 2: How Does the Human Body Deal With Glucose?

In a perfect world, our bodies digest glucose a few times each day. At the point when we eat, our bodies immediately start the most common way of handling glucose. With the assistance of the pancreas, chemicals start the breakdown of food substances. The pancreas, which produces chemicals like insulin, is pivotal to our body's glucose breakdown. At the point when we eat, our bodies signal the pancreas to deliver insulin to manage the developing glucose levels.

On the other hand, some people can't rely on their pancreas to do what it's supposed to do. At the point when the pancreas doesn't create insulin as it ought to, diabetes can occur. Individuals in this present circumstance need external support (insulin infusions) to process and oversee glucose in the body.

Insulin opposition is one more reason for diabetes, in which the liver neglects to perceive insulin in the body and keeps on delivering exorbitant measures of glucose.

The liver is a vital organ for the body's interaction with glucose since it helps to produce glucose on a regular basis. Free fatty acids are released from stored fat when the body does not produce enough insulin. Ketoacidosis is a condition that can result from this. Ketones, are substances created by the liver when fat is separated, and they pose danger to the body when present in large quantities.

## How Does Your Body Make Glucose?

It principally comes from food varieties rich in sugars, similar to bread, potatoes, and organic products. As you eat, food makes a trip down your throat to your stomach. There, acids and proteins separate it into little pieces. During that cycle, glucose is delivered. It goes into your digestive organs where it is consumed. From that point, it passes into your circulatory system. Once in the blood, insulin assists glucose with getting to your cells, and that is precisely how you get glucose into your circulatory system.

Glucose, or blood sugar, is a basic sort of sugar. Your body's daily functions can be affected if your blood sugar levels fall too low (hypoglycemia) or rise too high (hyperglycemia).

Glucose is the least complex sort of carbohydrate (carb), making it a monosaccharide, signifying "one sugar." Different monosaccharides incorporate fructose, galactose, and ribose. Here, dietary glucose and different sugars in the long run convert to blood glucose in the body.

Alongside fat and protein, glucose is one of the body's essential fuel sources.

Individuals can get glucose from complex carbs, for example, earthy colored rice, oats, vegetables, and so on, and also from basic carbs, for example, white bread, pasta, table sugar, etc. Based on how quickly the body digests the sugar, carbs are categorized as simple or complex. It is common knowledge that the body digests complex carbs more slowly and that they provide a more stable source of energy. As a result, they are the healthier choice. The effects of unmanaged glucose levels may be severe and last a lifetime.

## How does the body interact with glucose?

Your body preferably utilizes glucose on numerous occasions a day.

At the point when you eat, it rapidly begins attempting to deal with glucose and different starches. After that, with assistance from the pancreas, enzymes begin to break them down.

The pancreas, which produces chemicals like insulin, is fundamental for how your body manages glucose.

At the point when you eat, your body causes the pancreas to deliver insulin to deal with the rising glucose level. Muscle, fat, and other different cells then, at that point, use glucose for energy or store it as fat for some time in the future. When the pancreas does not produce insulin as it should, diabetes may develop. For this situation, you might require outside help (insulin infusions) to process and control glucose in the body.

Insulin resistance can also cause diabetes. This is the point at which the body's cells don't detect insulin, and a lot of sugar stays in the circulation system.

At the point when the body doesn't answer insulin how it ought to, it prevents glucose from entering your body cells and being utilized for energy. Your cells respond by signaling the production of ketones, which takes place at night, or when you fast or eat less.

On the long-haul, with insulin obstruction, your insulin levels might turn out to be low. Your body may likewise separate fat from fat cells. While, the liver continues delivering more ketones, bringing your blood pH down to an acidic level.

As a result, the development of ketones and changes in blood pH might become risky.. This occasion is known as ketoacidosis. It is an extreme state of diabetes that requires quick clinical treatment.

## Ketogenic diet and diabetes

The keto diet has acquired ubiquity, however, it's a clinical eating routine which is quite unpredictable.

As indicated by a recent report, a low-carb or keto diet might lessen body weight, yet individuals with diabetes and taking specific drugs might have an expanded unpredictable rate experiencing ketoacidosis.

Other negative effects which may affect others, includes high cholesterol, which is linked to cardiovascular disease. Before beginning any diet plan, it is best to discuss it with your doctor to help prevent complications.

## What Food Varieties Are High In Glucose?

Food is changed over into energy by our body. People gain energy and calories from glucose, protein, and fat. Although, carbohydrates are the main energy source for our body system. Carbs are switched over completely to glucose, a type of sugar, in our bodies. Numerous foods contain fat, protein, and carbohydrates. How quickly our bodies convert feasts into glucose is impacted by how much of these are present in each food we eat.

Here is an illustration of what various food varieties mean for our glucose levels:

## Starch

Bread, rice, pasta, potatoes, vegetables, organic products, sugar, yogurt, and milk all contain carbohydrates.

Our bodies convert each of the sugars we consume into glucose. This quickly affects our glucose levels, in the span of a little while of eating.

## Protein

Fish, meat, cheddar cheese, and peanut butter are completely remembered for proteins. Even though our bodies convert some piece of the protein we consume into glucose. Most of this is put away in our liver as opposed to being delivered into the circulation system. Protein utilization affects glucose levels in the body on a minor scale.

## Fat

Margarine, salad dressing, avocado, and olive oil are completely remembered for fats. We convert less than 10% of the fat we consume into glucose. The sugar in fat is gradually processed and doesn't prompt an ascent in glucose.

Indeed, even while fat doesn't give a lot of glucose, a high-fat eating regimen can influence how rapidly our bodies digest starches.

Fat represses the processing of carbs, which thus postpones the ascent in glucose levels. This can bring about an ascent in glucose a few hours after eating. Some people might be surprised by this delayed reaction. Before heading to sleep, an individual could have a glucose perusing that is near typical after having a high-fat supper. However, the following morning, their fasting blood sugar may exceed 200. This is because the carbs in the dinner took the body the entire sleeping time for it to be processed.

The most fundamental thing to recollect is that eating dinners containing protein, carbs, and a humble piece of fat can assist with keeping up with glucose levels from going excessively high or excessively fast.

## Is Glucose Destructive To Our Bodies?

A high blood sugar level for an extended period can result in serious health issues if left untreated.

Hyperglycemia harms the blood vessels that supply blood to significant organs. It can likewise raise the risk of coronary illness, stroke, kidney sickness, vision issues, and nerve issues.

These issues seldom show up in youngsters or teens, or in the people who have recently had the illness for a couple of years. Notwithstanding, grown-ups with diabetes can experience it, particularly if their diabetes has not been successfully overseen or controlled.

When your blood sugar level is higher than your normal range, hyperglycemia (high blood sugar) may be a possibility. Your diabetes medical care group will illuminate you about your objective levels. A solitary high glucose estimation isn't commonly the justification for concern. It occurs to people with diabetes more often. You could consider changing your insulin or feast plans.

In any case, you could disapprove of your hardware, for example, in a case when your insulin injector is not working. At any rate, seek immediate medical attention to regain control of your blood sugar levels.

# Chapter 3: The blessing of having a balanced blood sugar level

I'll give it a hundred-to-one shot that you're like the 93% of Americans who are metabolically undesirable, and balancing out your blood glucose can be an incredible asset for assuming command over your well-being. While glucose adjustment isn't a fix-all, your blood glucose is associated with all of your organ frameworks and, subsequently, contacts all pieces of your well-being here and there.

From your emotional wellness to your weight, your sexual coexistence to your bedtime — there's a connection to blood glucose, which is the reason balancing your levels is an amazing asset.

With the present circumstances, how precisely does adjusting your glucose work on your well-being?

# Here are 4 long-term advantages of balancing your blood glucose;

## 1. Invert insulin opposition

We've gabbed about dysregulated glucose adding to the improvement of insulin obstruction, which is firmly connected with weight, elevated cholesterol, high fatty substances, and the advancement of persistent circumstances like prediabetes, and cardiovascular sickness. High glucose fluctuation makes your body work harder (produce more insulin) to keep glucose in range, which worsens insulin opposition and damages your well-being. Adding more insulin and more glucose creates a vicious cycle.

Turning around insulin obstruction is urgent to keeping away from conditions like T2D, stoutness, prediabetes, and glucose intolerance. It might likewise assist with moderating circumstances like PCOS in women, persistent exhaustion, and incendiary problems like rheumatoid joint inflammation.

While insulin opposition is mind-boggling and influences numerous substantial frameworks, ongoing studies and research recommends that the three most remarkable instruments for switching it are exercise, diet, and bringing down glucose levels.

At the core of switching your insulin obstruction is settling your blood glucose and utilizing these four mainstays of well-being which includes; nourishment, exercise, rest, and stress control in order to keep your blood glucose in range.

## 2. Improved healthspan

Healthspan is the time of your life spent healthy. Obesity, insulin resistance, and poor glycemic control are all metabolic-related conditions that can result in major age-related diseases like cancer, diabetes, heart disease, stroke, and high blood pressure. Studies have additionally connected insulin protection to mind well-being, which is pivotal to life span and the counteraction of mental degradation.

Research in diabetic patients have shown changes in cerebrum design and capability connected to the advancement of diabetes, as well as changes in neurons related to energy balance. This indicates that insulin obstruction and its aggravation to diabetes can cause degradation to the mind and this results in a decrease in general mental wellbeing, which is intently attached to healthspan.

Insulin obstruction and the waistline size have additionally been demonstrated to be related to the shortening of white blood cell telomeres, which is characteristic of maturing in age.

This proposes that insulin opposition and expanded waistline size adds to diminishing life and health span.

Maintaining a healthy blood glucose range can help you live a longer life because uncontrollable glucose level contributes to insulin resistance.

## 3. Further develop chemical wellbeing

Assuming your blood glucose is messed up, it can affect your endocrine framework, which produces chemicals.

Consider endocrines as chemical substance couriers in the body that guide specific cells. The body's systems begin to fail when hormones are tampered with.

Blood glucose levels can have an impact on a wide range of hormones, including those related to organ function, insulin resistance, sex hormones, hormones that control appetite, and stress hormones.

In women, insulin resistance has been linked to a decrease in estrogen production, which may raise the risk of certain cancers, such as breast and ovarian cancer.

High blood glucose is likewise connected with expanded degrees of cortisol, a pressure chemical that, when raised after some time, can add to irritation, weight gain, and related metabolic diseases. By keeping your blood glucose stable, you can uphold the strength of your chemicals and, thus, your major real frameworks.

## 4. Manage weight

Insulin resistance is linked to high glucose variability (frequent peaks and valleys) and elevated fasting glucose; both of which can make it more difficult to lose weight and cause unwanted weight gain.

Late examination has shown that insulin flagging and the capability of carrier proteins that are driven by insulin are diminished in those with more fat tissue, regardless of whether they have typical blood glucose levels.

In a similar vein, individuals who had previously been obese or overweight but had lost weight showed higher levels of insulin sensitivity, indicating that their insulin resistance was reduced as a result of their weight loss.

Making healthier choices regarding your diet, exercise routine, sleeping schedule, and stress management strategies is necessary for stabilizing and maintaining blood glucose levels.

At the point when you center around holding blood glucose levels in line, your natural information from your blood glucose levels steers you to better food decisions. The over-restriction and binge-eating cycle that frequently causes people to regain their weight despite their best efforts can be avoided by making healthier food choices and exercising at the right times to reverse insulin resistance.

On the flip side of the coin, here are four short-term advantages of maintaining stable blood glucose levels Maintaining stable glucose levels is essential to long-term health and avoiding the onset of chronic conditions. However, shouldn't something be said about the present moment? What advantages should be expected in the initial or beginning stages of balancing your blood glucose levels?

## 1. Stabilized energy, reduced attention deficit

Raised blood glucose — high fasting glucose, or because of a dinner high in refined carbs — can prompt an inclination to drowsy, exhausted, or give you cerebrum haze. You can avoid the afternoon slump and reap the benefits of sustained energy when your blood glucose levels are well-controlled and your insulin sensitivity is raised.

## 2. Improved Aura

Research has connected high glycemic fluctuation, explicitly occurrences of glucose spikes and valleys, with sensations of crabbiness, uneasiness, and stress.

Low blood glucose levels have been linked to feelings of nervousness in many diabetic patient studies, while high blood glucose levels have been linked to feelings of frustration and agitation.

Keeping glucose in check and forestalling outrageous changes can assist with overseeing emotional episodes and keep you more ready and playful as opposed to battling pessimistic sentiments and irritability.

### 3. Fewer cravings

When you consume foods high in refined carbohydrates, your blood glucose rises, triggering an excessive production of insulin to cope. When the insulin overproduction gets up to speed, your glucose crashes, driving you to hunger for something sweet to bring your blood glucose level up to ordinary levels, and the cycle proceeds.

Indeed, even lenient low blood glucose (between 60-80 mg/dL) expanded the drive for hyper-attractive, fatty food varieties. By getting your blood glucose under tight restraints, you can get off the glucose rollercoaster and better control your desires.

## 4. Better skin

A spike in blood glucose causes an ascent in insulin levels, which can build the creation of sex chemicals called androgens, which are connected to the wellbeing of the skin.

At the point when insulin levels are high, androgens lead to the expanded creation of sebum and keratinocytes, which can leave skin feeling thick and slick and lead to undesirable breakouts. Studies have shown that having a low glycemic diet can result in a decrease in skin breakout issues.

# Conclusion

Similarly, as with numerous ailments, it's simpler to manage glucose issues before they get out of hand.. Also, balanced glucose levels are crucial for keeping your body working at its ideal.

A nutritious, balanced diet, enhanced with work out sessions, are essential for counteraction and treatment plans when accessible. For certain individuals, however, this isn't sufficient.

Individuals with diabetes might experience difficulty keeping up with solid and steady glucose levels. Assuming that you're living with diabetes, intently observing your glucose levels is a viable method for keeping away from inconveniences.

Dealing with your diabetes might be quite tasking however it's worth the work.

Your overall health is linked to your blood glucose levels. Balancing your blood glucose levels can improve your mood, sleep quality, sexual life, concentration, and other aspects of your life.